The Super-Mediterranean

The Definitive Guide to Start Cooking with Amazing Mediterranean Recipes

Raphael Chapman

Table of contents

3

European Posole

Preparation Time: 10 minutes

Cooking Time: 25 minutes

Servings: 2

Ingredients:

- 1 ½ cup water
- 6 oz chicken fillet
- 1 chili pepper, chopped
- 1 onion, diced
- 1 tsp. butter
- ½ tsp. salt
- ½ tsp. paprika
- 1 tbsp. fresh dill, chopped

Directions:

1. Pour water in the saucepan.
2. Add chicken fillet and salt. Boil it for 15 minutes over the medium heat.
3. Then remove the chicken fillet from water and shred it with the help of the fork.
4. Return it back in the hot water.
5. Melt butter in the skillet and add diced onion. Roast it until light brown and transfer in the shredded chicken.
6. Add paprika, dill, chili pepper, and mix up.
7. Close the lid and simmer Posole for 5 minutes.

Nutrition:

Calories 207,

Fat 8.3 g,

Carbs 6 g,

Protein 25.4 g

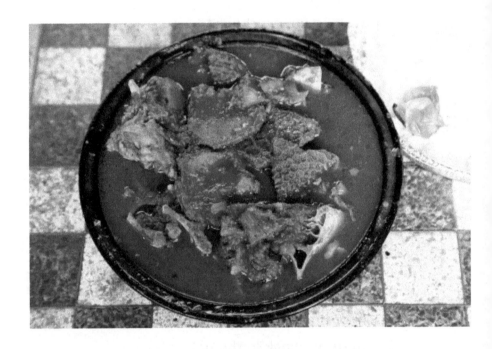

Mango Chicken Salad

Preparation Time: 10 minutes

Cooking Time: 12 minutes

Servings: 3

Ingredients:

- 1 cup lettuce, chopped
- 1 cup arugula, chopped
- 1 mango, peeled, chopped
- 8 oz chicken breast, skinless, boneless
- 1 tbsp. lime juice
- 1 tsp. sesame oil
- ½ tsp. salt
- ½ tsp. ground black pepper
- 1 tsp. butter

Directions:

1. Sprinkle the chicken breast with salt and ground black pepper.
2. Melt butter in the skillet and add chicken breast.
3. Roast it for 10 minutes over the medium heat. Flip it on another side from time to time.
4. Meanwhile, combine together lettuce, arugula, mango, and sesame oil in the salad bowl.
5. Add lime juice.
6. Chop the cooked chicken breast roughly and chill it to the room temperature.
7. Add it in the mango salad and mix up.

Nutrition:

Calories 183,

Fat 5.2 g,

Carbs 17.4 g,

Protein 17.2 g

Chicken Zucchini Boats

Preparation Time: 15 minutes

Cooking Time: 30 minutes

Servings: 2

Ingredients:

- 1 zucchini
- ½ cup ground chicken
- ½ tsp. chipotle pepper
- ½ tsp. tomato sauce
- 1 oz Swiss cheese, shredded
- ½ tsp. salt
- 4 tbsp. water

Directions:

1. Trim the zucchini and cut it on 2 halves.
2. Remove the zucchini pulp.
3. In the mixing bowl mix up together ground chicken, chipotle pepper, tomato sauce, and salt.
4. Fill the zucchini with chicken mixture and top with Swiss cheese.
5. Place the zucchini boats in the tray. Add water.
6. Bake the boats for 30 minutes at 355°F.

Nutrition:

Calories 134,

Fat 6.3 g,

Carbs: 7.1g

Protein 13.4 g

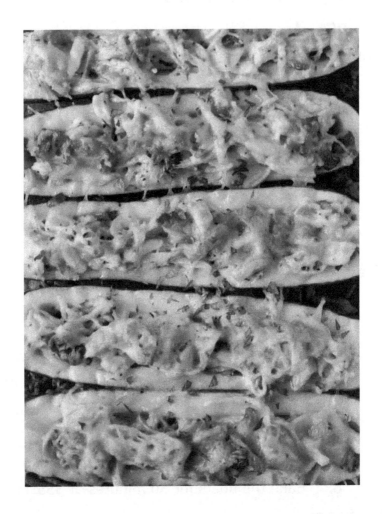

Urban Chicken Alfredo

Preparation Time: 10 minutes

Cooking Time: 20 minutes

Servings: 2

Ingredients:

- 1 onion, chopped
- 1 sweet red pepper, roasted, chopped
- 1 cup spinach, chopped
- ½ cup cream
- 1 tsp. cream cheese
- 1 tbsp. olive oil
- ½ tsp. ground black pepper
- 8 oz chicken breast, skinless, boneless, sliced

Directions:

1. Mix up together sliced chicken breast with ground black pepper and put in the saucepan.
2. Add olive oil and mix up.
3. Roast the chicken for 5 minutes over the medium-high heat. Stir it from time to time.
4. After this, add chopped sweet pepper, onion, and cream cheese.
5. Mix up well and bring to boil.
6. Add spinach and cream. Mix up well.
7. Close the lid and cook chicken Alfredo for 10 minutes more over the medium heat.

Nutrition:

Calories 279,

Fat 14 g,

Carbs: 6.9 g

Protein 26.4 g

Tender Chicken Quesadilla

Preparation Time: 10 minutes

Cooking Time: 20 minutes

Servings: 4

Ingredients:

- 2 bread tortillas
- 1 tsp. butter
- 2 tsp. olive oil
- 1 tsp. Taco seasoning
- 6 oz chicken breast, skinless, boneless, sliced
- 1/3 cup Cheddar cheese, shredded
- 1 bell pepper, cut on the wedges

Directions:

1. Pour 1 tsp. of olive oil in the skillet and add chicken.
2. Sprinkle the meat with Taco seasoning and mix up well.
3. Roast chicken for 10 minutes over the medium heat. Stir it from time to time.
4. Then transfer the cooked chicken in the plate.
5. Add remaining olive oil in the skillet.
6. Then add bell pepper and roast it for 5 minutes. Stir it all the time.
7. Mix up together bell pepper with chicken.
8. Toss butter in the skillet and melt it.
9. Put 1 tortilla in the skillet.

10. Put Cheddar cheese on the tortilla and flatten it.
11. Then add chicken-pepper mixture and cover it with the second tortilla.
12. Roast the quesadilla for 2 minutes from each side.
13. Cut the cooked meal on the halves and transfer in the serving plates.

Nutrition:

Calories 167,

Fat 8.2 g,

Carbs 16.4 g,

Protein 24.2 g

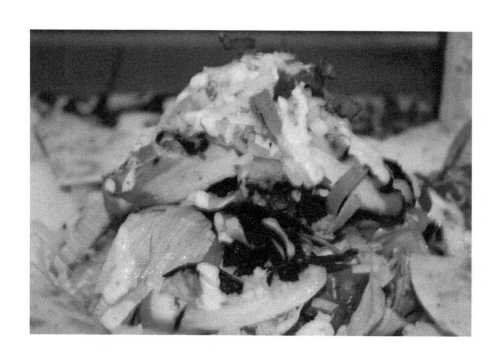

Light Caesar

Preparation Time: 10 minutes

Cooking Time: 10 minutes

Servings: 4

Ingredients:

- 4 oz chicken fillet, chopped
- ¼ cup black olives, chopped
- 2 cups lettuce, chopped
- 1 tbsp. mayo sauce
- 1 tsp. lemon juice
- ½ oz Parmesan cheese, shaved
- 1 tsp. olive oil
- ½ tsp. ground black pepper
- ½ tsp. coconut oil

Directions:

1. Sprinkle the chicken fillet with ground black pepper.
2. Heat up coconut oil and add chopped chicken fillet.
3. Roast it got 10 minutes or until it is cooked. Stir it from time to time.
4. Meanwhile, mix up together black olives, lettuce, Parmesan in the bowl.
5. Make mayo dressing: whisk together mayo sauce, olive oil, and lemon juice.
6. Add the cooked chicken in the salad and shake well.
7. Pour the mayo sauce dressing over the salad.

Nutrition:

Calories 134,

Fat 13.3 g,

Carbs 2 g,

Protein 9.4 g

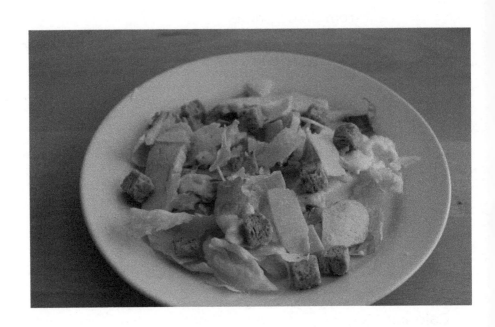

Chicken Parm

Preparation Time: 10 minutes

Cooking Time: 30 minutes

Servings: 4

Ingredients:

- 4 chicken steaks (4 oz each steak)
- ½ cup crushed tomatoes
- ¼ cup fresh cilantro
- 1 garlic clove, diced
- ½ cup of water
- 1 onion, diced
- 1 tsp. olive oil
- 3 oz Parmesan, grated
- 3 tbsp. Panko breadcrumbs
- 2 eggs, beaten
- 1 tsp. ground black pepper

Directions:

1. Pour olive oil in the saucepan.
2. Add garlic and onion. Roast the vegetables for 3 minutes.
3. Then add fresh cilantro, crushed tomatoes, and water.
4. Simmer the mixture for 5 minutes.

5. Meanwhile, mix up together ground black pepper and eggs.
6. Dip the chicken steaks in the egg mixture.
7. Then coat them in Panko breadcrumbs and again in the egg mixture.
8. Coat the chicken steaks in grated Parmesan.
9. Place the prepared chicken steaks in the crushed tomato mixture.
10. Close the lid and cook chicken parm for 20 minutes. Flip the chicken steaks after 10 minutes of cooking.
11. Serve the chicken parm with crushed tomatoes sauce.

Nutrition:

Calories 354,

Fat 21.3 g,

Carbs 12 g,

Protein 32.4 g

Chicken Bolognese

Preparation Time: 7 minutes

Cooking Time: 25 minutes

Servings: 4

Ingredients:

- 1 cup ground chicken
- 2 oz Parmesan, grated
- 1 tbsp. olive oil
- 2 tbsp. fresh parsley, chopped
- 1 tsp. chili pepper
- 1 tsp. paprika
- ½ tsp. dried oregano
- ¼ tsp. garlic, minced
- ½ tsp. dried thyme
- 1/3 cup crushed tomatoes

Directions:

1. Heat up olive oil in the skillet.

2.   Add ground chicken and sprinkle it with chili pepper, paprika, dried oregano, dried thyme, and parsley. Mix up well.

3.   Cook the chicken for 5 minutes and add crushed tomatoes. Mix up well.

4.   Close the lid and simmer the chicken mixture for 10 minutes over the low heat.

5.   Then add grated Parmesan and mix up.

6.   Cook chicken bolognese for 5 minutes more over the medium heat.

Nutrition:

Calories 154,

Fat 9.3 g,

Carbs 6 g,

Protein 15.4 g

Jerk Chicken

Preparation Time: 10 minutes

Cooking Time: 30 minutes

Servings: 2

Ingredients:

- 2 chicken thighs, skinless, boneless
- 1 tsp. fresh ginger, chopped
- 1 garlic clove, chopped
- ½ spring onion, chopped
- 1 tsp. liquid honey
- 1 tsp. fresh parsley, chopped
- 1 tsp. fresh coriander, chopped
- ¼ tsp. chili flakes
- ¼ tsp. ground black pepper
- 2 tsp. lemon juice

Directions:

1. Mix up together fresh ginger, garlic, onion, liquid honey, parsley, coriander, chili flakes, and ground black pepper.
2. Rub the chicken thighs with honey mixture generously.
3. Preheat the grill to 385°F.
4. Place the chicken thighs in the grill and cook for 30 minutes. Flip the chicken thighs on another side after 15 minutes of cooking. The cooked jerk chicken should have a brown crust.
5. Sprinkle the cooked chicken with lemon juice.

Nutrition:

Calories 139,

Fat 7.3 g,

Carbs 4 g,

Protein 19.4 g

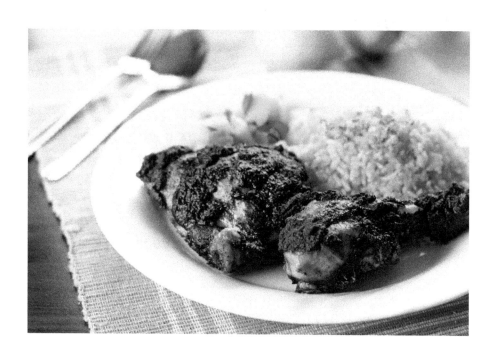

Crack Chicken

Preparation Time: 10 minutes

Cooking Time: 30 minutes

Servings: 4

Ingredients:

- 4 chicken thighs, skinless, boneless
- 1 tsp. ground black pepper
- ½ tsp. salt
- 1 tsp. paprika
- ¼ cup Cheddar cheese, shredded
- 1 tbsp. cream cheese
- ½ tsp. garlic powder
- 1 tsp. fresh dill, chopped
- 1 tbsp. butter
- 1 tsp. olive oil
- ½ tsp. ground nutmeg

Directions:

1. Grease the baking dish with butter.
2. Then heat up olive oil in the skillet.

3. Meanwhile, rub the chicken thighs with ground nutmeg, garlic powder, paprika, and salt. Add ground black pepper.

4. Roast the chicken thighs in the hot oil over the high heat for 2 minutes from each side.

5. Then transfer the chicken thighs in the prepared baking dish.

6. Mix up together Cheddar cheese, cream cheese, and dill.

7. Top every chicken thigh with cheese mixture and bake for 25 minutes at 365°F.

Nutrition:

Calories 79,

Fat 7.3 g,

Carbs 1 g,

Protein 2.4 g

Pomegranate Chicken Thighs

Preparation Time: 10 minutes

Cooking Time: 10 minutes

Servings: 2

Ingredients:

- 1 tbsp. pomegranate molasses
- 8 oz chicken thighs (4 oz each chicken thigh)
- ½ tsp. paprika
- 1 tsp. cornstarch
- ½ tsp. chili flakes
- ½ tsp. ground black pepper
- 1 tsp. olive oil
- ½ tsp. lime juice

Directions:

1. In the shallow bowl mix up together ground black pepper, chili flakes, paprika, and cornstarch.
2. Rub the chicken thighs with spice mixture.
3. Heat up olive oil in the skillet.
4. Add chicken thighs and roast them for 4 minutes from each side over the medium heat.
5. When the chicken thighs are light brown, sprinkle them with pomegranate molasses and roast for 1 minute from each side.

Nutrition:

Calories 374,

Fat 21.3 g,

Carbs 9 g,

Protein 30.4 g

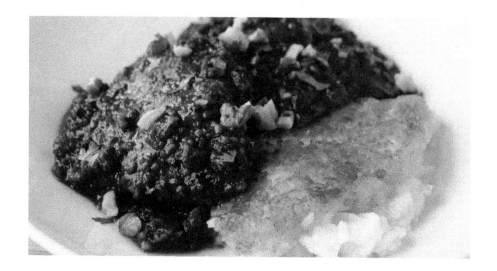

Butter Chicken

Preparation Time: 15 minutes

Cooking Time: 30 minutes

Servings: 5

Ingredients:

- 1-lb. chicken fillet
- 1/3 cup butter, softened
- 1 tbsp. rosemary
- ½ tsp. thyme
- 1 tsp. salt
- ½ lemon

Directions:

1. Churn together thyme, salt, and rosemary.
2. Chop the chicken fillet roughly and mix up with churned butter mixture.
3. Place the prepared chicken in the baking dish.
4. Squeeze the lemon over the chicken.
5. Chop the squeezed lemon and add in the baking dish.
6. Cover the chicken with foil and bake it for 20 minutes at 365°F.
7. Then discard the foil and bake the chicken for 10 minutes more.

Nutrition:

Calories 254,

Fat 19.3 g,

Carbs 1 g,

Protein 36.4 g

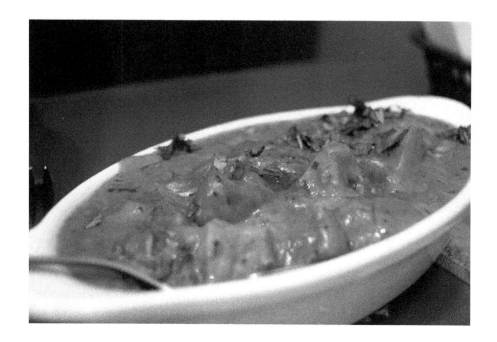

Santa le Skillet Chicken

Preparation Time: 10 minutes

Cooking Time: 20 minutes

Servings: 4

Ingredients:

- 12 oz chicken breast, skinless, boneless, chopped
- 1 tbsp. taco seasoning
- 1 tbsp. nut oil
- ½ tsp. cayenne pepper
- ½ tsp. salt
- ½ tsp. garlic, chopped
- ½ red onion, sliced
- 1/3 cup black beans, canned, rinsed
- ½ cup Mozzarella, shredded

Directions:

1. Rub the chopped chicken breast with taco seasoning, salt, and cayenne pepper.
2. Place the chicken in the skillet, add nut oil and roast it for 10 minutes over the medium heat. Mix

up the chicken pieces from time to time to avoid burning.

3. After this, transfer the chicken in the plate.
4. Add sliced onion and garlic in the skillet. Roast the vegetables for 5 minutes. Stir them constantly. Then add black beans and stir well. Cook the ingredients for 2 minute more.
5. Add the chopped chicken and mix up well. Top the meal with Mozzarella cheese.
6. Close the lid and cook the meal for 3 minutes.

Nutrition:

Calories 184,

Fat 6.3 g,

Carbs 13 g,

Protein 22.4 g

Tender Lamb Chops

Preparation Time: 10 minutes

Cooking Time: 6 hours

Servings: 8

Ingredients:

- 8 lamb chops
- ½ tsp. dried thyme
- 1 onion, sliced
- 1 tsp. dried oregano
- 2 garlic cloves, minced
- Pepper and salt

Directions:

1. Add sliced onion into the slow cooker.
2. Combine together thyme, oregano, pepper, and salt. Rub over lamb chops.
3. Place lamb chops in slow cooker and top with garlic.
4. Pour ¼ cup water around the lamb chops.
5. Cover and cook on low for 6 hours.
6. Serve and enjoy.

Nutrition:

Calories 140

Fat 9.9 g

Carbs 5.3 g

Protein 34 g

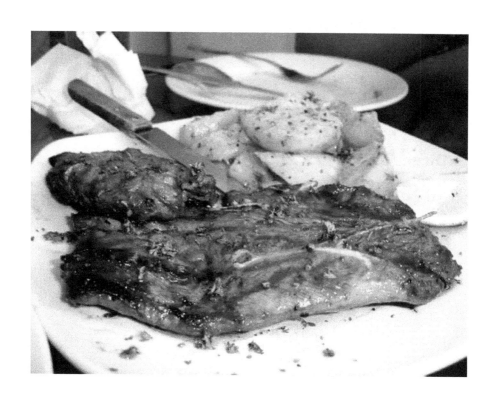

Smoky Pork & Cabbage

Preparation Time: 10 minutes

Cooking Time: 8 hours

Servings: 6

Ingredients:

- 3 lbs pork roast
- 1/2 cabbage head, chopped
- 1 cup water
- 1/3 cup liquid smoke
- 1 tbsp. kosher salt

Directions:

1. Rub pork with kosher salt and place into the crock pot.
2. Pour liquid smoke over the pork. Add water.
3. Cover and cook on low for 7 hours.
4. Remove pork from crock pot and add cabbage in the bottom of crock pot.
5. Place pork on top of the cabbage.
6. Cover again and cook for 1 hour more.
7. Shred pork with a fork and serve.

Nutrition:

Calories 484

Fat 21.5 g

Carbs 9g

Protein 66 g

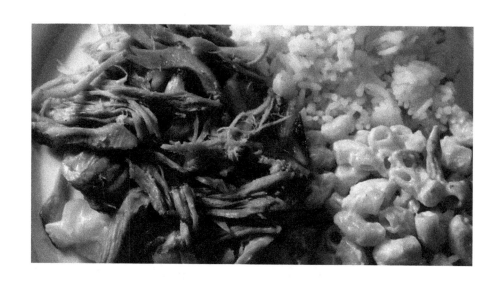

Seasoned Pork Chops

Preparation Time: 10 minutes

Cooking Time: 4 hours

Servings: 4

Ingredients:

- 4 pork chops
- 2 garlic cloves, minced
- 1 cup chicken broth
- 1 tbsp. poultry seasoning
- 1/4 cup olive oil
- Pepper and salt

Directions:

1. In a bowl, whisk together olive oil, poultry seasoning, garlic, broth, pepper, and salt.
2. Pour olive oil mixture into the slow cooker then place pork chops to the crock pot.
3. Cover and cook on high for 4 hours. Serve and enjoy.

Nutrition:

Calories 386

Fat 32.9 g

Carbs 3 g

Protein 20 g

Beef Stroganoff

Preparation Time: 10 minutes

Cooking Time: 8 hours

Servings: 2

Ingredients:

- 1/2 lb beef stew meat
- 10 oz mushroom soup, homemade
- 1 medium onion, chopped
- 1/2 cup sour cream
- 2.5oz mushrooms, sliced
- Pepper and salt

Directions:

1. Add all ingredients except sour cream into the crock pot and mix well.
2. Cover and cook on low for 8 hours.
3. Add sour cream and stir well.
4. Serve and enjoy.

Nutrition:

Calories 470

Fat 25 g

Carbs 8.6 g

Protein 49 g

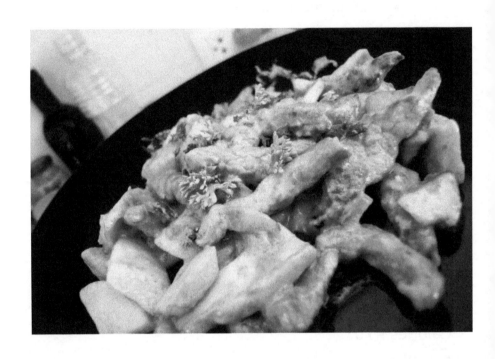

Lemon Beef

Preparation Time: 10 minutes

Cooking Time: 6 hours

Servings: 4

Ingredients:

- 1 lb beef chuck roast
- 1 fresh lime juice
- 1 garlic clove, crushed
- 1 tsp. chili powder
- 2 cups lemon-lime soda
- 1/2 tsp. salt

Directions:

1. Place beef chuck roast into the slow cooker.
2. Season roast with garlic, chili powder, and salt.
3. Pour lemon-lime soda over the roast.
4. Cover slow cooker with lid and cook on low for 6 hours. Shred the meat using fork.
5. Add lime juice over shredded roast and serve.

Nutrition:

Calories 355

Fat 16.8 g

Carbs 14 g

Protein 35.5 g

Herb Pork Roast

Preparation Time: 10 minutes

Cooking Time: 14 hours

Servings: 10

Ingredients:

- 5 lbs pork roast, boneless or bone-in
- 1 tbsp. dry herb mix
- 4 garlic cloves, cut into slivers
- 1 tbsp. salt

Directions:

1. Using a sharp knife make small cuts all over meat then insert garlic slivers into the cuts.
2. In a small bowl, mix together Italian herb mix and salt and rub all over pork roast.
3. Place pork roast in the crock pot.
4. Cover and cook on low for 14 hours.
5. Remove meat from crock pot and shred using a fork.
6. Serve and enjoy.

Nutrition:

Calories 327

Fat 8 g

Carbs 0.5 g

Protein 59 g

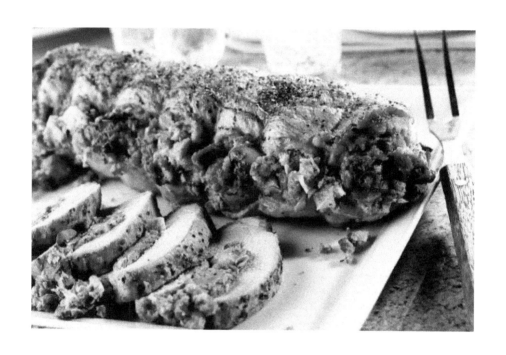

Greek Beef Roast

Preparation Time: 10 minutes

Cooking Time: 8 hours

Servings: 6

Ingredients:

- 2 lbs lean top round beef roast
- 1 tbsp. Italian seasoning
- 6 garlic cloves, minced
- 1 onion, sliced
- 2 cups beef broth
- ½ cup red wine
- 1 tsp. red pepper flakes
- Pepper
- Salt

Directions:

1. Season meat with pepper and salt and place into the crock pot.
2. Pour remaining ingredients over meat.
3. Cover and cook on low for 8 hours.
4. Shred the meat using fork.
5. Serve and enjoy.

Nutrition:

Calories 231

Fat 6 g

Carbs 4 g

Protein 35 g

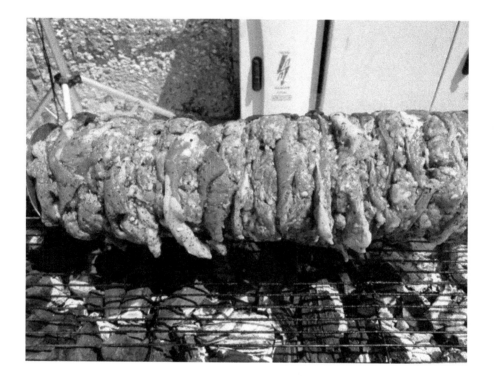

Tomato Pork Chops

Preparation Time: 10 minutes

Cooking Time: 6 hours

Servings: 4

Ingredients:

- 4 pork chops, bone-in
- 1 tbsp. garlic, minced
- ½ small onion, chopped
- 6 oz can tomato paste
- 1 bell pepper, chopped
- ¼ tsp. red pepper flakes
- 1 tsp. Worcestershire sauce
- 1 tbsp. dried Italian seasoning
- oz can tomatoes, diced
- 2 tsp. olive oil
- ¼ tsp. pepper
- 1 tsp. kosher salt

Directions:

1. Heat oil in a pan over medium-high heat.
2. Season pork chops with pepper and salt.
3. Sear pork chops in pan until brown from both the sides.
4. Transfer pork chops into the crock pot.
5. Add remaining ingredients over pork chops.
6. Cover and cook on low for 6 hours.
7. Serve and enjoy.

Nutrition:

Calories 325

Fat 23.4 g

Carbs 10 g

Protein 20 g

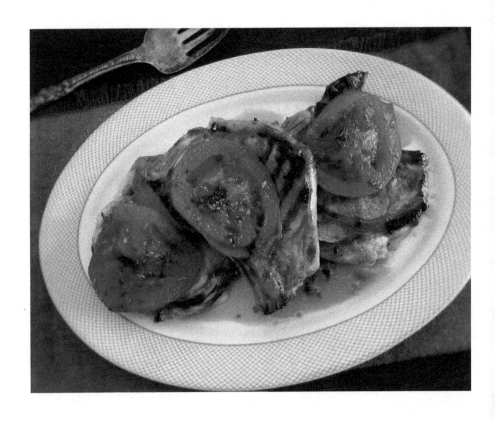

Greek Pork Chops

Preparation Time: 10 minutes

Cooking Time: 6 minutes

Servings: 8

Ingredients:

- 8 pork chops, boneless
- 4 tsp. dried oregano
- 2 tbsp. Worcestershire sauce
- 3 tbsp. fresh lemon juice
- ¼ cup olive oil
- 1 tsp. ground mustard
- 2 tsp. garlic powder
- 2 tsp. onion powder
- Pepper
- Salt

Directions:

1. Whisk together oil, garlic powder, onion powder, oregano, Worcestershire sauce, lemon juice, mustard, pepper, and salt.
2. Place pork chops in a baking dish then pour marinade over pork chops and coat well. Place in refrigerator overnight.
3. Preheat the grill.
4. Place pork chops on hot grill and cook for 3-4 minutes on each side.
5. Serve and enjoy.

Nutrition:

Calories 324

Fat 26.5 g

Carbs 2.5 g

Protein 18 g

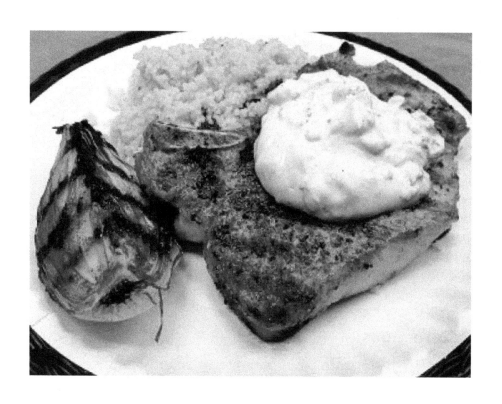

Pork Cacciatore

Preparation Time: 10 minutes

Cooking Time: 6 hours

Servings: 6

Ingredients:

- 1 ½ lbs pork chops
- 1 tsp. dried oregano
- 1 cup beef broth
- 3 tbsp. tomato paste
- 14 oz can tomatoes, diced
- 2 cups mushrooms, sliced
- 1 small onion, diced
- 1 garlic clove, minced
- 2 tbsp. olive oil
- ¼ tsp. pepper
- ½ tsp. salt

Directions:

1. Heat oil in a pan over medium-high heat.
2. Add pork chops in pan and cook until brown on both the sides.
3. Transfer pork chops into the crock pot.
4. Pour remaining ingredients over the pork chops.
5. Cover and cook on low for 6 hours.
6. Serve and enjoy.

Nutrition:

Calories 440

Fat 33 g

Carbs 6 g

Protein 28 g

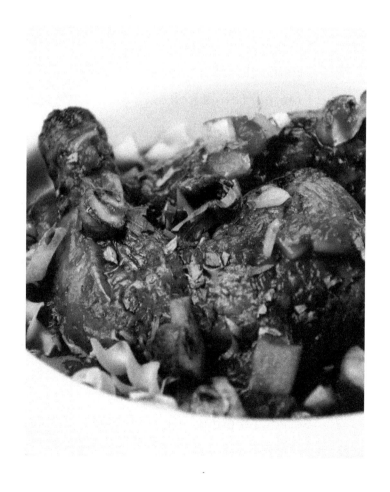

Pork with Tomato & Olives

Preparation Time: 10 minutes

Cooking Time: 30 minutes

Servings: 6

Ingredients:

- 6 pork chops, boneless and cut into thick slices
- 1/8 tsp. ground cinnamon
- 1/2 cup olives, pitted and sliced
- 8 oz can tomatoes, crushed
- 1/4 cup beef broth
- 2 garlic cloves, chopped
- 1 large onion, sliced
- 1 tbsp. olive oil

Directions:

1. Heat olive oil in a pan over medium-high heat.
2. Place pork chops in a pan and cook until lightly brown and set aside.
3. Cook garlic and onion in the same pan over medium heat, until onion is softened.
4. Add broth and bring to boil over high heat.
5. Return pork to pan and stir in crushed tomatoes and remaining ingredients.
6. Cover and simmer for 20 minutes.
7. Serve and enjoy.

Nutrition:

Calories 321

Fat 23 g

Carbs 7 g

Protein 19 g

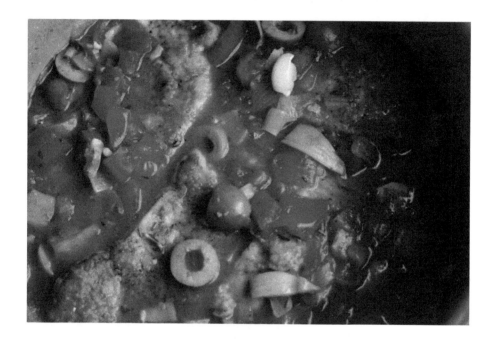

Pork Roast

Preparation Time: 10 minutes

Cooking Time: 1 hour 35 hours

Servings: 6

Ingredients:

- 3 lbs pork roast, boneless
- 1 cup water
- 1 onion, chopped
- 3 garlic cloves, chopped
- 1 tbsp. black pepper
- 1 rosemary sprig
- 2 fresh oregano sprigs
- 2 fresh thyme sprigs
- 1 tbsp. olive oil
- 1 tbsp. kosher salt

Directions:

1. Preheat the oven to 350°F.

2. Season pork roast with pepper and salt.

3. Heat olive oil in a stockpot and sear pork roast on each side, about 4 minutes.

4. Add onion and garlic. Pour in the water, oregano, and thyme and bring to boil for a minute.

5. Cover pot and roast in the preheated oven for 1 1/2 hours.

6. Serve and enjoy.

Nutrition:

Calories 502

Fat 23.8 g

Carbs 3 g

Protein 65 g

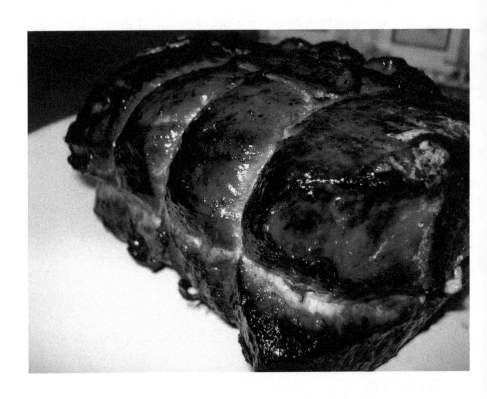

Easy Beef Kofta

Preparation Time: 10 minutes

Cooking Time: 10 minutes

Servings: 8

Ingredients:

- 2 lbs ground beef
- 4 garlic cloves, minced
- 1 onion, minced
- 2 tsp. cumin
- 1 cup fresh parsley, chopped
- ¼ tsp. pepper
- 1 tsp. salt

Directions:

1. Add all ingredients into the mixing bowl and mix until combined.
2. Roll meat mixture into the kabab shapes and cook in a hot pan for 4-6 minutes on each side or until cooked.
3. Serve and enjoy.

Nutrition:

Calories 223

Fat 7.3 g

Carbs 2.5 g

Protein 35 g

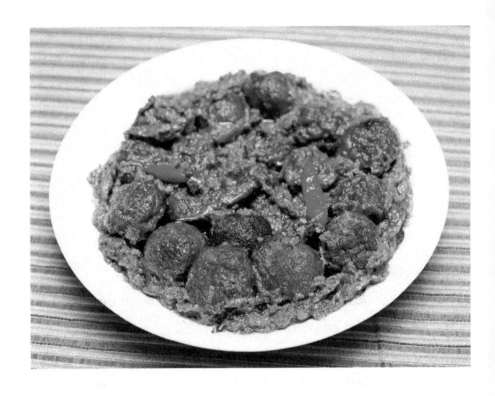

Lemon Pepper Pork Tenderloin

Preparation Time: 10 minutes

Cooking Time: 25 minutes

Servings: 4

Ingredients:

- 1 lb pork tenderloin
- 3/4 tsp. lemon pepper
- 2 tsp. dried oregano
- 1 tbsp. olive oil
- 3 tbsp. feta cheese, crumbled
- 3 tbsp. olive tapenade

Directions:

1.   Add pork, oil, lemon pepper, and oregano in a zip-lock bag and rub well and place in a refrigerator for 2 hours.
2.   Remove pork from zip-lock bag. Using sharp knife make lengthwise cut through the center of the tenderloin.
3.   Spread olive tapenade on half tenderloin and sprinkle with feta cheese.
4.   Fold another half of meat over to the original shape of tenderloin.
5.   Tie close pork tenderloin with twine at 2-inch intervals.
6.   Grill pork tenderloin for 20 minutes.
7.   Cut into slices and serve.

Nutrition:

Calories 215

Fat 9.1 g

Carbs 1 g

Protein 30.8 g

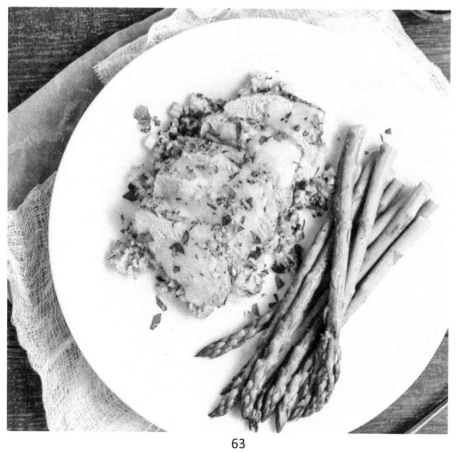

Cheese Pinwheels

Preparation Time: 20 minutes

Cooking Time: 25 minutes

Servings: 4

Ingredients:

- 1 tsp. chili flakes
- ½ tsp. dried cilantro
- 1 egg, beaten
- 1 tsp. cream cheese
- 1 oz Cheddar cheese, grated
- 6 oz pizza dough

Directions:

1. Roll up the pizza dough and cut into 6 squares.
2. Sprinkle the dough with dried cilantro, cream cheese, and Cheddar cheese.
3. Roll the dough in the shape of pinwheels, brush with beaten egg and bake in the preheated to 365°F oven for 25 minutes or until the pinwheels are light brown.

Nutrition: 16 Calories, 3.8g Protein, 12.1g Carbs, 11.2g Fat

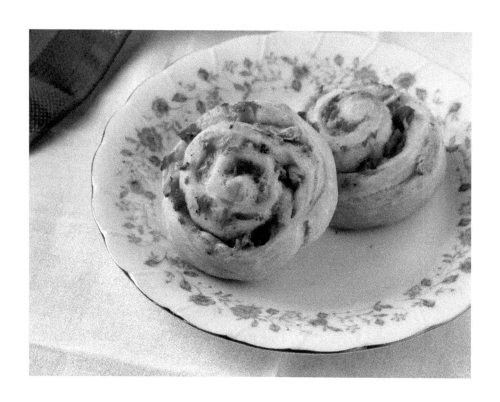

Ground Meat Pizza

Preparation Time: 15 minutes

Cooking Time: 35 minutes

Servings: 4

Ingredients:

- 7 oz ground beef
- 1 tsp. tomato paste
- ½ tsp. ground black pepper
- 2 egg whites, whisked
- ½ cup Mozzarella cheese, shredded
- 1 tsp. fresh basil, chopped

Directions:

1. Line the baking tray with baking paper. Preheat the oven to 370F.
2. Mix all ingredients except Mozzarella in the mixing bowl.
3. Then place the mixture in the tray and flatten it to get a thick layer.
4. Top the pizza with Mozzarella cheese and bake in the oven for 35 minutes.
5. Then cut the cooked pizza into the servings.

Nutrition: 213 Calories, 18g Protein, 17g Carbs, 12.8g Fat

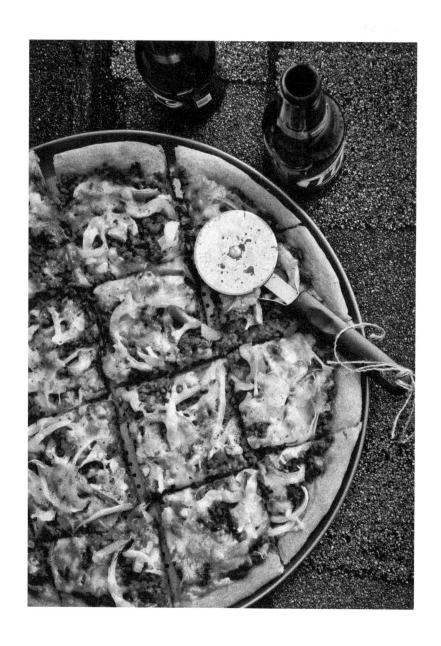

Quinoa Flour Pizza

Preparation Time: 15 minutes

Cooking Time: 15 minutes

Servings: 6

Ingredients:

- 1 oz pumpkin puree
- 3 tbsp. quinoa flour
- ½ tsp. dried oregano
- 1 cup Mozzarella cheese, shredded
- 1 tomato, chopped
- 1 tsp. olive oil

Directions:

1. Mix pumpkin puree, quinoa flour, and olive oil. Knead the dough.
2. Roll it up in the shape of pizza crust and transfer in the lined with a baking paper baking tray.
3. Then top the pizza crust with tomato, oregano, and Mozzarella cheese.
4. Bake the pizza at 365°F for 15 minutes.

Nutrition: 38 Calories, 2g Protein, 10g Carbs, 8g Fat

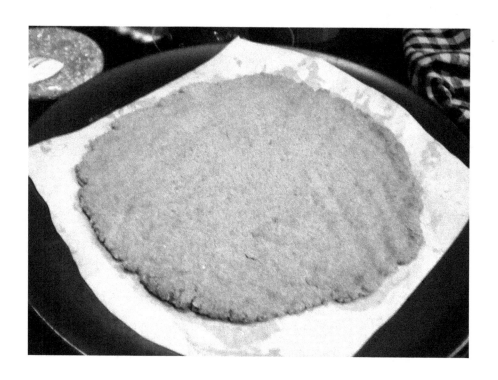

Greek Style Bread with Black Olives

Preparation Time: 25 minutes

Cooking Time: 45 minutes

Servings: 12

Ingredients:

- 1 cup black olives, pitted, sliced
- 1 tbsp. avocado oil
- ½ oz fresh yeast
- 4 oz cream cheese
- 2 cup wheat flour, whole grain
- 3 eggs, beaten
- 1 tsp. olive oil, melted
- 1 tsp. sugar

Directions:

1. In the big bowl combine fresh yeast, sugar, and cream cheese. Stir it until yeast is dissolved.
2. Then add olive oil and eggs. Stir the dough mixture until homogenous and add 1 cup of wheat flour. Mix it up until smooth.
3. Add olives and remaining flour. Add avocado oil and knead the non-sticky dough.
4. Transfer the dough into the non-sticky dough mold.

5. Cook the bread for 65 minutes at 350°F.

6. When the bread is cooked, cool it well and remove it from the mold.

7. Slice the bread.

Nutrition: 176 Calories, 6.6g Protein, 27g Carbs, 4.6g Fat

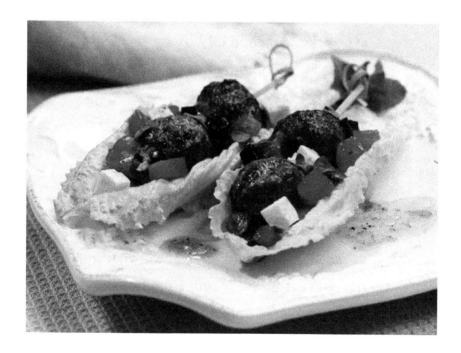

Turkey Flatbread

Preparation Time: 15 minutes

Cooking Time: 30 minutes

Servings: 8

Ingredients:

- 1 ½ cup ground turkey
- 1 tsp. baking powder
- ¼ cup plain yogurt
- 9 oz wheat flour, whole grain
- 1 tsp. avocado oil
- 1 tsp. tomato paste

Directions:

1. Make the yeast dough: mix baking powder, plain yogurt, and whole-grain flour.
2. Knead the non-sticky dough and leave it in a warm place for 15 minutes.
3. After this, roll up the dough in the shape of a square and transfer it in the lined baking tray.
4. Bake it at 365°F for 10 minutes.
5. Meanwhile, mix ground turkey, tomato paste, and avocado oil.
6. Spread the ground turkey mixture over the flatbread and bake it at 365f for 20 minutes more.

Nutrition: 246 Calories,20.7g Protein, 25.8g Carbs, 7.3g Fat

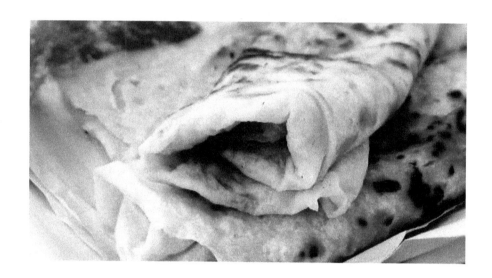

Pepper Flatbread Bites

Preparation Time: 20 minutes

Cooking Time: 10 minutes

Servings: 8

Ingredients:

- 2 tbsp. olive oil, softened
- 1/3 cup plain yogurt
- 9 oz wheat flour, whole grain
- 1 tsp. olive oil
- 1 cup bell pepper, chopped
- 1 oz Parmesan, grated

Directions:

1. Mix olive oil and plain yogurt.
2. Then add flour and knead the soft dough.
3. Cut the dough into 8 pieces and roll into the rounds.
4. Then preheat olive oil in the skillet.
5. Put the dough rounds in the skillet and roast for 3 minutes per side.
6. Then top the cooked dough bites with bell pepper and Parmesan.
7. Cook the meal with closed lid for 2 minutes.

Nutrition: 174 Calories, 5.2g Protein, 26.3g Carbs, 5.2g Fat

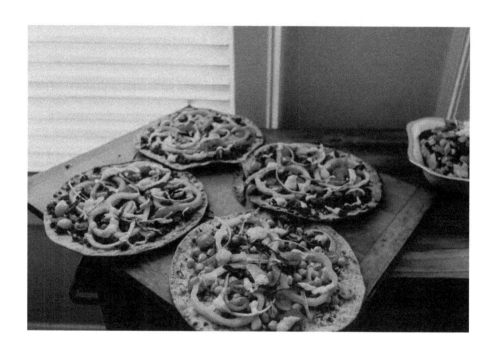

Artichoke Pizza

Preparation Time: 15 minutes

Cooking Time: 15 minutes

Servings: 4

Ingredients:

- 7 oz pizza crust
- 5 oz artichoke hearts, canned, drained, chopped
- 1 tsp. fresh basil, chopped
- 1 tomato, sliced
- 1 cup Monterey Jack cheese, shredded

Directions:

1. Line the pizza mold with baking paper.
2. Then put the pizza crust inside.
3. Top it with sliced tomato, canned artichoke hearts, and basil.
4. Then top the pizza with Monterey Jack cheese and transfer in the preheated to 365°F oven.
5. Cook the pizza for 20 minutes.

Nutrition: 247 Calories, 12.1g Protein, 28.2g Carbs, 10.2g Fat

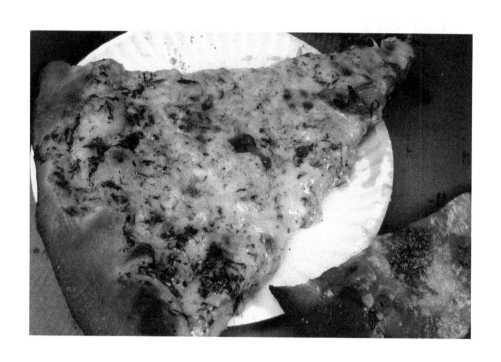

3-Cheese Pizza

Preparation Time: 15 minutes

Cooking Time: 10 minutes

Servings: 6

Ingredients:

- 1 pizza crust, cooked
- ½ cup Mozzarella, shredded
- ½ cup Cheddar cheese, shredded
- 2 oz Parmesan, grated
- ¼ cup tomato sauce
- 1 tsp. Italian seasonings

Directions:

1. Put the pizza crust in the baking pan.
2. Then brush it with tomato sauce and Italian seasonings.
3. After this, sprinkle the pizza with Mozzarella, Cheddar cheese, and Parmesan.
4. Bake the pizza for 10 minutes at 375°F.

Nutrition: 106 Calories, 7g Protein, 6.3g Carbs, 6.1g Fat

Chickpea Pizza

Preparation Time: 10 minutes

Cooking Time: 25 minutes

Servings: 4

Ingredients:

- 4 tbsp. marinara sauce
- 7 oz pizza dough
- 1 tomato, sliced
- 1 red onion, sliced
- 5 oz chickpeas, canned
- ½ cup Mozzarella cheese, shredded

Directions:

1. Roll up the pizza dough in the shape of pizza crust and transfer in the pizza mold.
2. Then brush the pizza crust with marinara sauce and sprinkle with sliced onion, tomato, and chickpeas.
3. Top the chickpeas with mozzarella cheese and bake the pizza for 25 minutes at 355°F.

Nutrition: 266 Calories, 7.6g Protein, 31.9g Carbs, 12.4g Fat

Arugula Fig Chicken

Preparation Time: 15 minutes

Cooking Time: 30 minutes

Servings: 4

Ingredients :

- 2 tsp. cornstarch
- 2 clove garlic, crushed
- ¾ cup Mission figs, chopped
- ¼ cup black or green olives, chopped
- 1 bag baby arugula
- ½ cup chicken broth
- 8 skinless chicken thighs
- 2 tsp. olive oil
- 2 tsp. brown sugar
- ½ cup red wine vinegar
- Ground black pepper and salt, to taste

Directions:

1. Over medium stove flame, heat the oil in a skillet or saucepan (preferably of medium size).
2. Add the chicken, sprinkle with some salt and cook until evenly brown. Set it aside.
3. Add and sauté the garlic.

4. In a mixing bowl, combine the vinegar, broth, cornstarch and sugar. Add the mixture into the pan and simmer until the sauce thickens.

5. Add the figs and olives; simmer for a few minutes. Serve warm with chopped arugula on top.

Nutrition:

Calories – 364

Fat – 14g

Carbs – 29g

Protein – 31g

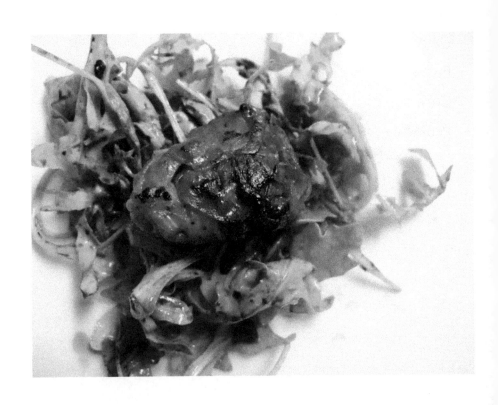

Parmesan Chicken Gratin

Preparation Time: 10 minutes

Cooking Time: 30 minutes

Servings: 4

Ingredients:

- 2 chicken thighs, skinless, boneless
- 1 tsp. paprika
- 1 tbsp. lemon juice
- ½ tsp. chili flakes
- ¼ tsp. garlic powder
- 3 oz Parmesan, grated
- 1/3 cup milk
- 1 onion, sliced
- 2 oz pineapple, sliced

Directions:

1. Chop the chicken thighs roughly and sprinkle them with paprika, lemon juice, chili flakes, garlic powder, and mix up well.
2. Arrange the chopped chicken thighs in the baking dish in one layer.
3. Then place sliced onion over the chicken.
4. Add the layer of sliced pineapple.
5. Mix up together milk and Parmesan and pour the liquid over the pineapple,

6. Cover the surface of the baking dish with foil and bake gratin for 30 minutes at 355°F.

Nutrition:

Calories 100,

Fat 5.2,

Carbs 6.7,

Protein 8.1

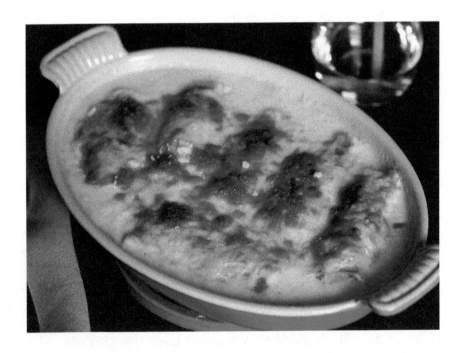

Chicken Saute

Preparation Time: 10 minutes

Cooking Time: 25 minutes

Servings: 2

Ingredients:

- 4 oz chicken fillet
- 4 tomatoes, peeled
- 1 bell pepper, chopped
- 1 tsp. olive oil
- 1 cup of water
- 1 tsp. salt
- 1 chili pepper, chopped
- ½ tsp. saffron

Directions:

1. Pour water in the pan and bring it to boil.
2. Meanwhile, chop the chicken fillet.
3. Add the chicken fillet in the boiling water and cook it for 10 minutes or until the chicken is tender.

4. After this, put the chopped bell pepper and chili pepper in the skillet.
5. Add olive oil and roast the vegetables for 3 minutes.
6. Add chopped tomatoes and mix up well.
7. Cook the vegetables for 2 minutes more.
8. Then add salt and a ¾ cup of water from chicken.
9. Add chopped chicken fillet and mix up.
10. Cook the saute for 10 minutes over the medium heat.

Nutrition:

Calories 192,

Fat 7.2 g,

Carbs 14.4 g,

Protein 19.2 g

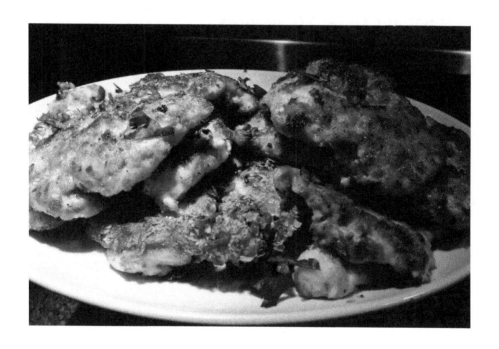

Grilled Marinated Chicken

Preparation Time: 35 minutes

Cooking Time: 20 minutes

Servings: 6

Ingredients:

- 2-lb. chicken breast, skinless, boneless
- 2 tbsp. lemon juice
- 1 tsp. sage
- ½ tsp. ground nutmeg
- ½ tsp. dried oregano
- 1 tsp. paprika
- 1 tsp. onion powder
- 2 tbsp. olive oil
- 1 tsp. chili flakes
- 1 tsp. salt
- 1 tsp. apple cider vinegar

Directions:

1. Make the marinade: whisk together apple cider vinegar, salt, chili flakes, olive oil, onion powder, paprika, dried oregano, ground nutmeg, sage, and lemon juice.
2. Then rub the chicken with marinade carefully and leave for 25 minutes to marinate.
3. Meanwhile, preheat grill to 385°F.
4. Place the marinated chicken breast in the grill and cook it for 10 minutes from each side.
5. Cut the cooked chicken on the servings.

Nutrition:

Calories 218

Fat 8.2 g,

Carbs 0.4 g,

Protein 32.2 g

Chicken Fillets with Artichoke Hearts

Preparation Time: 10 minutes

Cooking Time: 30 minutes

Servings: 3

Ingredients:

- 1 can artichoke hearts, chopped
- 12 oz chicken fillets (3 oz each fillet)
- 1 tsp. avocado oil
- ½ tsp. ground thyme
- ½ tsp. white pepper
- 1/3 cup water
- 1/3 cup shallot, roughly chopped
- 1 lemon, sliced

Directions:

1. Mix up together chicken fillets, artichoke hearts, avocado oil, ground thyme, white pepper, and shallot.
2. Line the baking tray with baking paper and place the chicken fillet mixture in it.
3. Then add sliced lemon and water.
4. Bake the meal for 30 minutes at 375°F. Stir the ingredients during cooking to avoid burning.

Nutrition:

Calories 267,

Fat 8.2 g,

Carbs 10.4 g,

Protein 35.2 g

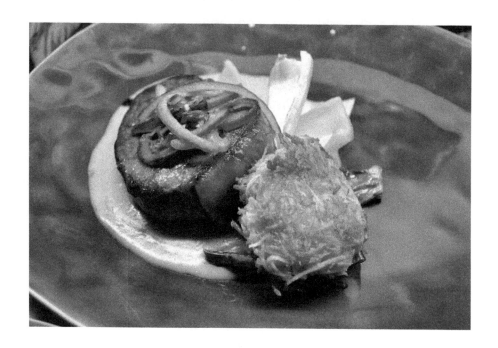

Chicken Loaf

Preparation Time: 10 minutes

Cooking Time: 40 minutes

Servings: 4

Ingredients:

- 2 cups ground chicken
- 1 egg, beaten
- 1 tbsp. fresh dill, chopped
- 1 garlic clove, chopped
- ½ tsp. salt
- 1 tsp. chili flakes
- 1 onion, minced

Directions:

1. In the mixing bowl combine together all ingredient and mix up until you get smooth mass.
2. Then line the loaf dish with baking paper and put the ground chicken mixture inside.
3. Flatten the surface well.
4. Bake the chicken loaf for 40 minutes at 355°F.
5. Then chill the chicken loaf to the room temperature and remove from the loaf dish. Slice it.

Nutrition:

Calories 167,

Fat 6.2 g,

Carbs 3.4 g,

Protein 32.2 g

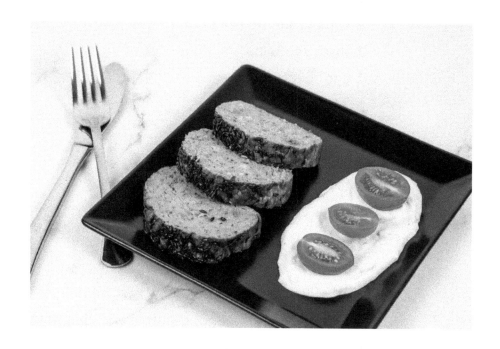

Chicken Meatballs with Carrot

Preparation Time: 10 minutes

Cooking Time: 10 minutes

Servings: 8

Ingredients:

- 1/3 cup carrot, grated
- 1 onion, diced
- 2 cups ground chicken
- 1 tbsp. semolina
- 1 egg, beaten
- ½ tsp. salt
- 1 tsp. dried oregano
- 1 tsp. dried cilantro
- 1 tsp. chili flakes
- 1 tbsp. coconut oil

Directions:

1. In the mixing bowl combine together grated carrot, diced onion, ground chicken, semolina, egg, salt, dried oregano, cilantro, and chili flakes.
2. With the help of scooper make the meatballs.
3. Heat up the coconut oil in the skillet.
4. When it starts to shimmer, put meatballs in it.
5. Cook the meatballs for 5 minutes from each side over the medium-low heat.

Nutrition:

Calories 107,

Fat 4.2 g,

Carbs 4.6 g,

Protein 11.2 g

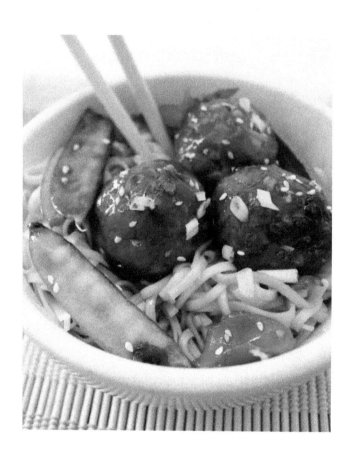

Chicken Burgers

Preparation Time: 15 minutes

Cooking Time: 15 minutes

Servings: 4

Ingredients:

- 8 oz ground chicken
- 1 cup fresh spinach, blended
- 1 tsp. minced onion
- ½ tsp. salt
- 1 red bell pepper, grinded
- 1 egg, beaten
- 1 tsp. ground black pepper
- 4 tbsp. Panko breadcrumbs

Directions:

1. In the mixing bowl mix up together ground chicken, blended spinach, minced garlic, salt, grinded bell pepper, egg, and ground black pepper.
2. When the chicken mixture is smooth, make 4 burgers from it and coat them in Panko breadcrumbs.
3. Place the burgers in the non-sticky baking dish or line the baking tray with baking paper.
4. Bake the burgers for 15 minutes at 365F.
5. Flip the chicken burgers on another side after 7 minutes of cooking.

Nutrition:

Calories 177,

Fat 5.2 g,

Carbs 10.4 g,

Protein 13.2 g

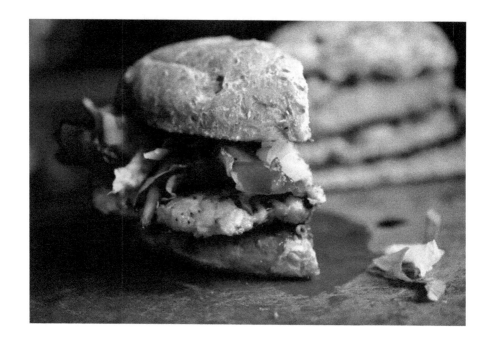

Duck Patties

Preparation Time: 15 minutes

Cooking Time: 10 minutes

Servings: 8

Ingredients:

- 1-lb. duck breast, skinless, boneless
- 1 tsp. semolina
- ½ tsp. cayenne pepper
- 2 eggs, beaten
- 1 tsp. salt
- 1 tbsp. fresh cilantro, chopped
- 1 tbsp. olive oil

Directions:

1. Chop the duck breast on the tiny pieces (grind it) and combine together with semolina, cayenne pepper, salt, and cilantro. Mix up well.
2. Then add eggs and stir gently.
3. Pour olive oil in the skillet and heat it up.
4. Place the duck mixture in the oil with the help of the spoon to make the shape of small patties.
5. Roast the patties for 3 minutes from each side over the medium heat.
6. Then close the lid and cook patties for 4 minutes more over the low heat.

Nutrition:

Calories 106,

Fat 5.2 g,

Carbs 6.2 g,

Protein 13.2 g

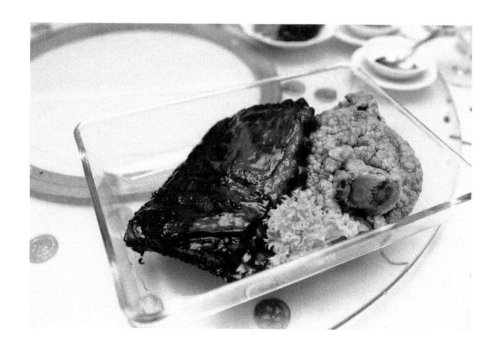

Creamy Chicken Pate

Preparation Time: 2 hours

Cooking Time: 20 minutes

Servings: 6

Ingredients:

- 8 oz chicken liver
- 3 tbsp. butter
- 1 white onion, chopped
- 1 bay leaf
- 1 tsp. salt
- ½ tsp. ground black pepper
- ½ cup of water

Directions:

1. Place the chicken liver in the saucepan.
2. Add onion, bay leaf, salt, ground black pepper, and water.
3. Mix up the mixture and close the lid.

4. Cook the liver mixture for 20 minutes over the medium heat.
5. Then transfer it in the blender and blend until smooth.
6. Add butter and mix up until it is melted.
7. Pour the pate mixture in the pate ramekin and refrigerate for 2 hours.

Nutrition:

Calories 322,

Fat 18.2 g,

Carbs 12.7 g,

Protein 19.2 g

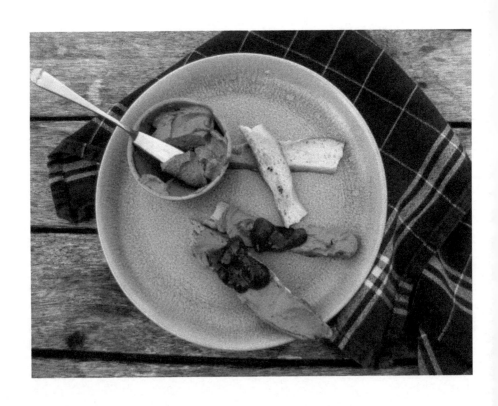

Curry Chicken Drumsticks

Preparation Time: 10 minutes

Cooking Time: 30 minutes

Servings: 4

Ingredients:

- 4 chicken drumsticks
- 1 apple, grated
- 1 tbsp. curry paste
- 4 tbsp. milk
- 1 tsp. coconut oil
- 1 tsp. chili flakes
- ½ tsp. minced ginger

Directions:

1. Mix up together grated apple, curry paste, milk, chili flakes, and minced garlic.
2. Put coconut oil in the skillet and melt it.
3. Add apple mixture and stir well.
4. Then add chicken drumsticks and mix up well.
5. Roast the chicken for 2 minutes from each side.
6. Then preheat oven to 360°F.
7. Place the skillet with chicken drumsticks in the oven and bake for 25 minutes.

Nutrition:

Calories 152,

Fat 7.2 g,

Carbs 9.4 g,

Protein 13.2 g

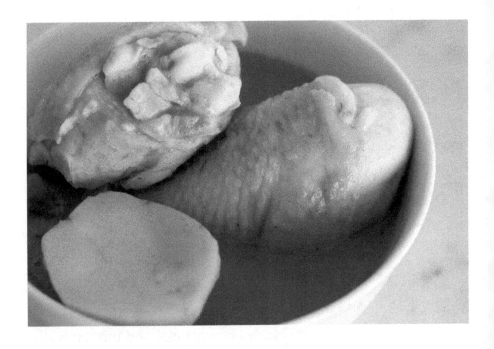

Chicken Enchiladas

Preparation Time: 20 minutes

Cooking Time: 15 minutes

Servings: 5

Ingredients:

- 5 corn tortillas
- 10 oz chicken breast, boiled, shredded
- 1 tsp. chipotle pepper
- 3 tbsp. green salsa
- ½ tsp. minced garlic
- ½ cup cream
- ¼ cup chicken stock
- 1 cup Mozzarella, shredded
- 1 tsp. butter, softened

Directions:

1. Mix up together shredded chicken breast, chipotle pepper, green salsa, and minced garlic.
2. Then put the shredded chicken mixture in the center of every corn tortilla and roll them.
3. Spread the baking dish with softened butter from inside and arrange the rolled corn tortillas.
4. Then pour chicken stock and cream over the tortillas.
5. Top them with shredded Mozzarella.
6. Bake the enchiladas for 15 minutes at 365°F.

Nutrition:

Calories 152,

Fat 5.2 g,

Carbs 16.5 g,

Protein 19.6 g

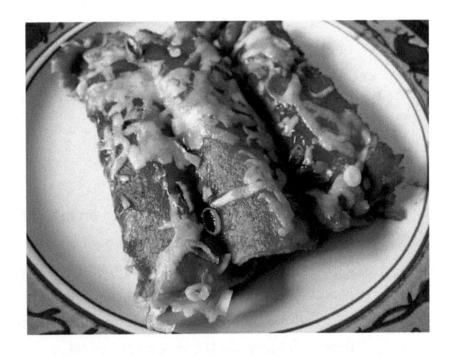

Chicken Fajitas

Preparation Time: 15 minutes

Cooking Time: 15 minutes

Servings: 2

Ingredients:

- 1 bell pepper
- ½ red onion, peeled
- 5 oz chicken fillets
- 1 garlic clove, sliced
- 1 tbsp. olive oil
- 1 tsp. balsamic vinegar
- 1 tsp. chili pepper
- ½ tsp. salt
- 1 tsp. lemon juice
- 2 flour tortillas

Directions:

1. Cut the bell pepper and chicken fillet on the wedges.

2. Then slice the onion.

3. Pour olive oil in the skillet and heat it up.

4. Add chicken wedges and sprinkle them with chili pepper and salt.

5. Roast the chicken for 4 minutes. Stir it from time to time.

6. After this, add lemon juice and balsamic vinegar. Mix up well.

7. Add bell pepper, onion, and garlic clove.

8. Roast fajitas for 10 minutes over the medium-high heat. Stir it from time to time.

9. Put the cooked fajitas on the tortillas and transfer in the serving plates.

Nutrition:

Calories 346,

Fat 14.2 g,

Carbs 23.4 g,

Protein 25.2 g

Chicken Stroganoff

Preparation Time: 10 minutes

Cooking Time: 20 minutes

Servings: 4

Ingredients:

- 1 cup cremini mushrooms, sliced
- 1 onion, sliced
- 1 tbsp. olive oil
- ½ tsp. thyme
- 1 tsp. salt
- 1 cup Plain yogurt
- 10 oz chicken fillet, chopped

Directions:

1. Heat up olive oil in the saucepan.
2. Add mushrooms and onion.
3. Sprinkle the vegetables with thyme and salt. Mix up well and cook them for 5 minutes.
4. After this, add chopped chicken fillet and mix up well.
5. Cook the ingredients for 5 minutes more.
6. Then add plain yogurt, mix up well, and close the lid.
7. Cook chicken stroganoff for 10 minutes over the low heat.

Nutrition:

Calories 224,

Fat 9.2 g,

Carbs 7.4 g,

Protein 24.2 g

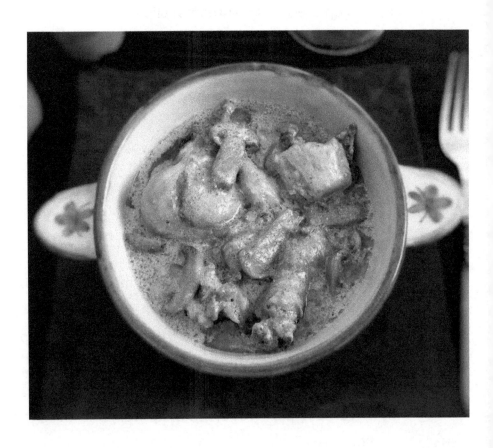

Lightning Source UK Ltd.
Milton Keynes UK
UKHW020706130521
383649UK00005B/78